Baking

Simple And Affordable Recipes For Fresh, Aromatic, And Tasty Bread And Bakery Products

(The Essential Cookbook For Everyone To Prepare Homemade Kneaded Bread)

Desmond Millington

TABLE OF CONTENT

Chapter 1: Baking Soda For Home: Impressive Application Of Baking Soda In The Home 1

Chapter 2: Gluten-Free Baked Goods: The Gluten-Free Cheat Food Concept 8

Chapter 4: Tenderization Of Meat 16

Chapter 5: Why Is Making Bread A Wise Decision? 20

Almond Sugar Cookies 40

Mexican Sweet Biscuits 42

Bean Roll-Ups 51

Classic Nut Date Moist Bread 53

Zucchini Brownies 57

Easily Remove Just Cool Just Take Just Cool Crunchy Cinnamon-Sugar Snacks 59

Cauliflower Cheesecake 61

Opera Cake 63

Scones 68

Easy Chocolate Molten Cakes 70

Almond Brownies 73

A Chocolate, Peanut Butter, And Banana Icebox Cake. 74

Coconut Crepe Cake 77

Vegan Oatmeal Cookies 80

Ingredients 80

Directions 81

Brownies With A Peanut Butter Twist 83

Bread Made With A Variety Of Whole Grains 86

Chapter 1: Baking Soda For Home: Impressive Application Of Baking Soda In The Home

Baking Soda Will Soon Replace Vinegar As The Remedy Of Choice For Common Kitchen Issues.

Baking Soda, Or Sodium Bicarbonate, Is One Of The Most Useful Ingredients For Cooking. In Addition To Its Common Use As A Leavening Agent In Baked Goods, Baking Soda Can Be Employed In The Kitchen For A Variety Of Unexpected Applications.

All Of Them Can Be Cleaned With Baking Soda, Including An Odorous Refrigerator, A Soiled Oven, And A Sheet Pan. In Addition, You May Be Surprised To Learn That Foods Such As Beans And Bagels May Benefit From The Addition Of Baking Soda If You're Looking For

Ways To Use Up That Box Of Baking Soda While Cooking.

The Baking Soda Can Be Used To Clean Your Priceless Cookware Without Causing Damage. If You Soak Them In Baking Soda For 2 10 To 20 Minutes, The Grease, Grime, And Food Will Be Effortlessly Removed.

Carpet Cleaner - To Effectively Eliminate Odours And Clean Your Carpet Without Endangering Your Children Or Pets, Use Baking Soda. Spread It Over Your Carpet And Vacuum It Up 2 10 To 20 Minutes Later.

Create A Natural Fruit And Vegetable Scrub By Combining A Teaspoon Of Water With A Teaspoon Of Salt. Using The Pastey Combination, Your Fruits And Vegetables Can Be Perfectly Cleaned Of Bacteria.

To Make A Paste For Cleaning Silverware, Combine Three Parts Baking Soda With One Part Water. Before Placing Your Silverware In A Large Dish Or Tray, It Should Be Coated In The Paste. After 2 10 To 20 Minutes, Rinse The Silverware Thoroughly.

Mix A Teaspoon Of Baking Soda With A Damp Sponge Or Rag To Clean Your Oven Without The Use Of Hazardous Chemicals. This Mixture Will Effectively Easily Remove Food And Grease.

The Combination Of Baking Soda And Vinegar Can Be Used To Clean A Drain. A Combination Of Vinegar And Baking Soda Is A Safer Alternative To The Hazardous Chemicals Commonly Used To Clean Drains. Following 2 10 Minutes Of Bubbling, The Mixture Is Rinsed With Hot Water. Just Wait Until You See How

Very Well Vinegar And Baking Soda Work For Cleaning!

Dishwasher Helper - Want To Find Out If Washing Dishes With Baking Soda Is Effective? Include It In Your Normal Dishwashing Cycle To Assist In Removing Grease And Grime From Plates.

In The Kitchen, Baking Soda Can Be Used As A Fire Extinguisher To Easily Put Out Small Grease Fires. It Should Quickly Extinguish A Small Pan Fire If Poured On It.

Can't Easily Remove That Foul Odour From Your Shoes. Consider Shoe Deodorizers. Deodorizing Shoes Is One Of The Numerous Common Uses For Baking Soda. Sprinkle Them Inside Your Shoes To Keep Them Smelling Fresh.

You Will Notice How Rapidly The Offensive Odour Vanishes.

Coffee And Tea Pot Cleaner - Combine One-Fourth Cup Of Baking Soda With One Quart Of Warm Water To Quickly Easily Remove Coffee Stains And Unpleasant Flavours From Your Coffee Or Teapot. Rub The Mixture Into And Onto Your Pots; If You Are Removing Stubborn Stains, Allow The Mixture To Sit For A Few Hours Before Rinsing.

Shower-Curtain Cleaner - To Eliminate Stains, Scrub Baking Soda Onto Your Shower Curtains. A Small Amount Of Water Will Quickly Easily Remove The Filth.

Easily Put A Box Or A Cup Of Baking Soda In Your Closet To Eliminate

Unpleasant Odours. To Keep Your Closet Smelling Clean And Fresh, Periodically Replace Its Contents.

Have You Ever Washed Your Car With Baking Soda? It Is The Ideal Component For The Ultimate Car Cleaning Because It Removes Grease And Grime With Ease. Combine 2 /8 Cup Baking Soda And 2 Cup Warm Water To Form A Paste. Before Rinsing, Apply The Paste To Your Vehicle's Tyres, Lights, Seats, And Glass Using A Sponge Or Rag. To Easily Remove Dirt And Grime From Your Paint, You Can Use A Gallon Of Baking Soda Diluted In Water. In Its Powdered Form, Baking Soda Is Abrasive; Therefore, Proper Dissolution Is Required.

Deodorizer For Cat Litter - Baking Soda Also Has Uses For Animals! Cover The Bottom Of The Litter Box With Baking

Soda, Then Fill It With Kitty Litter As Usual To Deodorise It Naturally. After Removing The Litre From The Box, Sprinkle Baking Soda On Top To Further Eliminate Odours.

Chapter 2: Gluten-Free Baked Goods: The Gluten-Free Cheat Food Concept

Ok, so last week you did not feel very well. You visited your doctor, underwent an examination, and a few days later received the most unexpected result: you have been diagnosed with celiac disease and are no longer permitted to consume gluten-containing foods. What will you do? (I'll likely grieve for a while until I begin to feel better again!). Does this imply that you cannot consume a slice of bread, a delicious cupcake, or a cookie for the rest of your life? The response is NO. There is still a way around this, and here is a cheat sheet to help you do so.

Your Expectations will only Cause You Pain —- Give up on it

Let's get straight to the point: gluten-free baking is completely different from regular baking. You will no longer mindlessly scoop a cup of flour from a 10 kg bag. Dear, the procedure has changed significantly.

For gluten-free dough to taste and feel like regular dough, for instance, it must have the consistency of pancake batter. Normal bakers will tell you it's wrong, but you're baking gluten-free now, so who cares? By adding more flour, the bread will become as hard as stone. And hitting someone on the head will likely result in their death!

Learn how to discard your previous habits and expectations now that you're baking gluten-free. Begin anew and be eager to discover new baking techniques. Sweep the gluten away from your kitchen. You are the "new" you, and you will no longer return to your old ways.

Combining Flours —- I adore your technique!

Don't allow yourself to get stuck with all-purpose gluten-free flour. Why? Because it is monotonous and there are numerous alternatives, including teff flour, rice flour, buckwheat flour, and others! Learn how to combine different types of gluten-free flour by conducting research. Try it in your baking and you'll notice the difference!

—- Baking by Weight Let's do some math!

Do you cherish math? If not, then proceed to spend time with each other. Most individuals are accustomed to baking in cups. That is fine. But what will you do if you run out of flour A while making a gluten-free family favourite cookie? You have available flour B and are aware that it can be substituted, but how much should you use? You cannot simply add another cup, correct? Invest in a small scale for your kitchen and learn to bake by weight. Thus, you will be able to accurately measure your ingredients, ensuring that your cookie, bread, or muffin will bake up very well. A few hours spent familiarising yourself with a conversion table won't hurt. Trust me. You'll be grateful later.

Everyone Makes Errors, so let's have some fun with it!

Do not expect to immediately master everything. That will only hurt you.

Allow yourself some time to master gluten-free baking. I am a firm believer of "practise makes perfect". A few errors along the way won't harm you; embrace them and learn from them. Discover, design, and bake! Feel the flour and decide which one you like. Learn how to create new mixtures and experiment with the batter and dough. Eventually, all things will come into the right place.

Chapter 3: Gluten-free Baked Goods Preparation

Are you prepared to bake incredible, mouthwatering gluten-free treats? Great! But before we proceed to the recipe section, let's discuss some essential kitchen preparations. Following these simple steps will make gluten-free baking safe, enjoyable, and worry-free.

Wash hands frequently and thoroughly.

Hand washing is always the first rule to follow. Making this a daily practise in the kitchen will help prevent food and cooking utensil contamination.

Clean the Dishes, Kitchen Utensils, and Counters.

Nonstick pans are easier to clean than traditional pans because there are typically no residues left behind. If possible, simply avoid using porous materials in the kitchen, such as wood or bamboo cutting boards. Gluten can adhere to the cracks and pores in these materials. When cleaning up spills or drying your hands, it is best to use disposable paper towels rather than fabric towels because fabric towels can also retain gluten.

Always Keep Your Kitchen Drawers Clean

Most silverware compartments are prone to crumbs. It is best to keep these drawers clean at all times. If you can afford it, gluten-free baking requires a separate set of cooking and baking tools. Easily put them in a separate drawer so they don't get mixed up with the rest of your cookware.

Store Individually

To prevent confusion and cross-contamination, store gluten-free foods in separate containers with the proper labels. Additionally, you can colour code them or use stickers to maintain order. Finally, designate a separate shelf or space in the refrigerator for gluten-free foods.

Gluten-Free Foods Are Priority

Do you intend to prepare two meals? If so, it is advisable to prepare gluten-free meals first. This is to ensure that none of the utensils, surfaces, cutting boards, etc. are contaminated.

Meals One at a Time

If possible, it is preferable to prepare each meal separately. Multitasking is extremely confusing, and the risk of cross-contamination is high.

Do Not Reuse

Do not fry gluten-free and regular foods in the same oil. Additionally, simply avoid using the same cooking water if you've used it to easy cook gluten-containing foods, such as pasta, previously.

Chapter 4: Tenderization Of Meat

The majority of cooks are accustomed to tenderising meat prior to cooking. This is done to save time during the cooking process. Additionally, this will aid in preserving the flavour of the food being cooked, as certain cooking ingredients may be sufficiently volatile. A case in point is the fact that sometimes only a small amount of liquid is required to make soup. However, this liquid could easily evaporate before the recipe's completion. This can occur when the meat requires additional time to become tender. Worst of all, some cooks would resort to adding additional water so that the boiling process would continue to tenderise the meat. When the first batch of water is drained, the majority of the meat and spice juices will have evaporated, rendering the overall dish tasteless. To prevent this from occurring, most cooks utilise meat tenderization techniques. This will not only preserve the flavour of the meat during cooking, but it can also reduce the cooking time.

Therefore, the question is what methods or processes are used to tenderise meat. There are numerous ways in which this can be accomplished. This can be accomplished through the use of tools, manual processes, or, in some cases, tenderising powder or baking soda.

Depending on what is most convenient for you, you may select any of the above options. Regarding the use of tools, you can always purchase a wood hammer or mallet for pounding the meat. This is typically done when the meat is thinly and uniformly sliced. Care must be taken so that the meat is not completely shredded during this process.

Others partially reheat the meat. They wish to bring the meat to a partially cooked state so that it will be easier to easy cook the meat quickly when necessary. Inadvertently bringing the meat to a state of complete tenderness will result in an unpleasant flavour, as spices have not yet been added in the majority of cases. If this method is the best option for you, you should choose it.

Marinating and adding spices can also make meat more tender and flavorful before cooking. This is the most common method for preparing meat specifically for the barbecue.

On the other hand, some individuals also employ the alkaline on the meat. Alkaline achieves this by altering the surface protein characteristics of meat. Still, it is recommended that the meat be sliced thinly so that baking soda can slowly penetrate the meat's surface. As for some individuals, they can add baking soda directly to the dish, but they must be cautious because this may affect the final flavour.

Chapter 5: Why Is Making Bread A Wise Decision?

You require it. Most people consume bread daily. Most individuals begin their day with some form of bread. A muffin or toast with your coffee and fresh egg s. In other countries, a baguette or chilaquiles may be available. In the majority of countries, lunch or dinner will include bread. Therefore, you must have it. Why not create it on your own? Previously, the excuse could have been that the task is time-consuming. With the invention of the home bread machine and the InstaPot, this justification is no longer valid. Here are the reasons why baking bread is a great idea.

It's nutritious

When you bake bread at home, you have control over the ingredients, allowing you to exclude gluten if you so choose. You can make it vegan. You can add seeds and grains, choose a flatbread, make it yeasty, or make it rise as baking powder or soda bread. You are in complete control of the bread. Oh, it feels so good to be in charge!

You can make it with wheat, whole wheat, white flour, or any of the other available grains. You possess options. If you only purchase store-bought items in the modern world, you have fewer options. Depending on the time of day, you may not even be able to purchase fresh items. But if you bake your own bread, you can guarantee that it will be fresh within a couple of hours. Whenever, day or night

Chapter 6: Small grain with significant potential as a superfood

In terms of nutritional value, oats are the highest quality grain grown in Central Europe. Consequently, this valuable grain is used in a number of the recipes in this book. Due to the fact that edible oats have been cultivated for approximately 7,000 years and have not undergone as many breeding changes as wheat or rye, for instance, some experts classify them as ancient grains.

Oats contain little gluten. This makes it appealing for a gluten-free diet. In baking, however, this is more of a disadvantage, as baked goods with a high oat content and low gluten content may lack stability and volume. For this reason, oats are used less frequently in industrially produced bread and are always supplemented with other, more gluten-rich cereals.

Most people are acquainted with oats in the form of oatmeal, as this is the most widely traded form. Oat flakes typically contain the entire grain, including both the outer layer and the seedling. Thus, vitamins, minerals, plant matter, and fibre are largely retained. Oatmeal is an excellent ingredient for baking. Tender oat flakes produce a more refined baked good than their heartier counterparts. If you prefer a finer consistency, you can further grind the oat flakes in the mixer before processing, resulting in a high-quality oat flour.

The essential amino acids in oats contribute to the growth of muscles, nerves, and chemical messengers. Fiber in the diet regulates digestion. In addition, oats are exceptionally high in protein for grains, containing approximately 2 2 percent protein. The protein content is primarily composed of the essential amino acids isoleucine, leucine, lysine, methionine, phenylalanine, and valine, which the body cannot produce on its own and must therefore obtain from an external source.

Isoleucine, leucine, and valine are required for the development and maintenance of muscle cells. Lysine is essential for growth, the production of enzymes, hormones, and antibodies, collagen synthesis, bone health, and tissue repair.

As a drug, methionine is used, among other things, to prevent kidney stones, to inhibit bacterial growth in cystitis, and as an ingredient in nutritional infusion solutions. In order to adequately supply the body with phenylalanine, which is required for the synthesis of important messenger substances, it must be consumed in large quantities, especially during times of stress.

In addition, oats contain the minerals magnesium, potassium, iron, calcium, phosphorus, and zinc, as very well as B vitamins and vitamin E. Due to their high fibre content, oats are regarded as a remedy for digestive issues. The grain's indigestible fibre forms a mucus film that protects the stomach and intestinal mucosa. In this manner, digestive issues and inflammation can be alleviated or cured. The high fibre content ensures that oats will keep you full for an extended period of time.

Due to its high fibre content, oat bran is a true miracle for weight loss: Due to its high fibre content, oat bran svery wells in the digestive tract and keeps you feeling full for a particularly long time. The fibre binds fats, which are then expelled undigested. In addition, they cleanse the intestines and help detoxify the body.

Chapter 7: Other Ingredients For Enjoyment Of Extremely Healthy Bread

Other popular grains and pseudo-grains for bread baking include buckwheat, corn, and millet. These grains are gluten-free and must therefore be combined with other grains. In general, it is beneficial to consume as many different types of grains as possible. Because each type of pseudo-grain contains very specific nutrients and ingredients, a particular variety is beneficial to the body. Particularly, the micronutrient content of certain pseudo-cereals is astoundingly high. Quinoa, amaranth, and others are not superfoods for anything!

Therefore, it is not only pleasurable and healthy to bake with a variety of ingredients and to try new things repeatedly! With a wide variety of foods, it is possible to achieve an optimal nutrient supply. Therefore, incorporate as many different grains as possible into your diet!

Nuts are the crunchiest delight in bread.

Nuts and almonds provide crispness and flavour to bread and rolls. Also, they are healthy. Their high content of essential omega-6 fatty acids is one reason. These play a vital role in nutrition because the body cannot produce them on its own and must be supplied with them. These fats are said to inhibit inflammatory responses and even protect against cancer.

Nuts are rich in antioxidants, or plant compounds that neutralise free radicals. In addition, Vitamin E is "coming cell protection." Nuts and almonds also have a prebiotic effect: They nourish beneficial intestinal bacteria, promoting a healthy intestinal flora and a strong immune system. Their high fibre content of up to 2 10 .2% makes nuts exceptionally nutritious bread ingredients!

The problem with nuts is their reputation as a fattening food. 2 00 grammes of walnuts, for instance, contain roughly 610 0 calories. However, research indicates that eating nuts can help you lose weight. How could this be? Due to the hard structure of the nut, which is not completely destroyed even when chewed, researchers believe that only a portion of the calories can be absorbed by the body. A significant portion is excreted undigested. In addition, studies indicate that nut consumption reduces cholesterol and maintains insulin levels. And a balanced insulin level means diminished appetite!

Kernels and seeds: a seduction with heightened potency

Kernels and seeds impart a hearty flavour to bread and have true superfood qualities. They contain everything a young plant needs to get off to a good start in life, so it is not surprising. They contain essential fatty acids as very well as vitamins E, A, and K. These can protect the body from inflammation. In addition, kernels are abundant in phytochemicals and omega-6 fatty acids, which are known for their beneficial effects on the cardiovascular system and blood vessels. They reduce the level of "bad" LDL cholesterol and prevent the absorption of a portion of the cholesterol in the diet.

Even more, they make you happy. Because the kernels contain arginine, an amino acid. This enlarges the blood vessels to improve blood circulation. Thus, the body is better supplied with oxygen, your general health improves, and you feel physically fit. They are also a good source of the amino acid tryptophan, which is a precursor to the happiness hormone serotonin. Absence of this messenger substance can result in susceptibility to stress, depression, and slowed cognitive performance.

The high fibre content of the kernels is an additional benefit. This will keep you satisfied for quite some time. Due to their high protein content, kernels are an excellent vegetable protein source.

Other popular grains and pseudo-grains for bread baking include buckwheat, corn, and millet. These grains are gluten-free and must therefore be combined with other grains. In general, it is beneficial to consume as many different types of grains as possible. Because each type of pseudo-grain contains very specific nutrients and ingredients, a particular variety is beneficial to the body. Particularly, the micronutrient content of certain pseudo-cereals is astoundingly high. Quinoa, amaranth, and others are not superfoods for anything!

Therefore, it is not only pleasurable and healthy to bake with a variety of ingredients and to try new things repeatedly! With a wide variety of foods, it is possible to achieve an optimal nutrient supply. Therefore, incorporate as many different grains as possible into your diet!

Nuts are the crunchiest delight in bread.

Nuts and almonds provide crispness and flavour to bread and rolls. Also, they are healthy. Their high content of essential omega-6 fatty acids is one reason. These play a vital role in nutrition because the body cannot produce them on its own and must be supplied with them. These fats are said to inhibit inflammatory responses and even protect against cancer.

Nuts are rich in antioxidants, or plant compounds that neutralise free radicals. In addition, Vitamin E is "coming cell protection." Nuts and almonds also have a prebiotic effect: They nourish beneficial intestinal bacteria, promoting a healthy intestinal flora and a strong immune system. Their high fibre content of up to 2 10 .2% makes nuts exceptionally nutritious bread ingredients!

The problem with nuts is their reputation as a fattening food. 2 00 grammes of walnuts, for instance, contain roughly 610 0 calories. However, research indicates that eating nuts can help you lose weight. How could this be? Due to the hard structure of the nut, which is not completely destroyed even when chewed, researchers believe that only a portion of the calories can be absorbed by the body. A significant portion is excreted undigested. In addition, studies indicate that nut consumption reduces cholesterol and maintains insulin levels. And a balanced insulin level means diminished appetite!

Kernels and seeds: a seduction with heightened potency

Kernels and seeds impart a hearty flavour to bread and have true superfood qualities. They contain everything a young plant needs to get off to a good start in life, so it is not surprising. They contain essential fatty acids as very well as vitamins E, A, and K. These can protect the body from inflammation. In addition, kernels are abundant in phytochemicals and omega-6 fatty acids, which are known for their beneficial effects on the cardiovascular system and blood vessels. They reduce the level of "bad" LDL cholesterol and prevent the absorption of a portion of the cholesterol in the diet.

Even more, they make you happy. Because the kernels contain arginine, an amino acid. This enlarges the blood vessels to improve blood circulation. Thus, the body is better supplied with oxygen, your general health improves, and you feel physically fit. They are also a good source of the amino acid tryptophan, which is a precursor to the happiness hormone serotonin. Absence of this messenger substance can result in susceptibility to stress, depression, and slowed cognitive performance.

The high fibre content of the kernels is an additional benefit. This will keep you satisfied for quite some time. Due to their high protein content, kernels are an excellent vegetable protein source.

Chapter 8: The Most Efficient Bread making Method

If you've never heated homemade bread before, consider the following advice:

Make sure TO FULLY KNEAD

The following seven-minute recipe is very well worth the effort! Don't skimp on the massaging time, as it contributes to enhancing the flavour and exterior of the bread.

THE WEATHER MAY AFFECT YOUR INGREDIENTS.

Assuming you live in a humid environment, it's likely that you'll need an additional 2 /8 to 1 cup of flour in addition to the recommended amount. Especially after the initial ascent, bread dough should be sticky, yet cohesive. As you work, the batter should come together and pull away from the sides of the bowl, leaving the bowl in good condition. I generally intend to have the actual lower portion of the mixture adhered to the bowl. Do whatever it takes to simply avoid adding too much flour, as the bread will become denser otherwise. Some of the batter will stick to your fingers when you first receive it. After the initial increase, it will be less difficult to manage!

Temperature influences how long it takes bread to rise.

If your home is cool, your bread will require additional time to rise. In the winter, when my home is typically cooler than usual, I turn the stove on for two to three minutes, then turn it off and let the bowl of batter rise inside. It is the ideal air for the rising batter that the broiler retains the heat for an extended period.

Simply avoid overworking the dough.

Do whatever it takes to simply avoid going off the deep end after the initial rise of your bread. Typically, I shape and manipulate my mixture for about a minute before returning it to the dish to rest for the second ascent. I prefer to have the container rise in the oven during the second rise so that I don't have to worry about moving the risen mixture. When it has fully risen, I simply ignite the stove and set the timer!

HOW MAY YOU DETERMINE IF BREAD IS COMPLETELY BAKED?

I enjoy using food thermometers. The sophistication of mine makes it extremely simple to use. The temperature of fully baked bread will be between 2 90 and 200 degrees Fahrenheit. Milk-based bread recipes should bake until 200 degrees, but since this one does not, I easily remove it when it reaches 2 90 degrees. The surface will be bright brown.

Almond Sugar Cookies

Ingredients:

- 2 pinch cardamom powder
- 2 teaspoon baking powder
- 1 cup butter

- 2 cup almond flour
- 1/2 cup granulated sugar
- 1/2 cup chopped almonds
- 2 pinch salt

Directions:

1. Spread wax paper on a baking sheet.
2. Sift together the almond flour, cardamom, salt, and baking powder.
3. In a separate bowl, cream the granulated sugar with the butter.
4. Add the ingredients that have been sifted. Fold dough together.
5. Refrigerate it for 20 minutes, 35 minutes, to 40 minutes.

6. Roll and cut the dough into a star shape.
7. Almonds chopped and sprinkled on top.
8. Bake between 15 and 20 minutes. After 45 to 50 minutes, serve.

Mexican Sweet Biscuits

Ingredients:

- 1 teaspoon salt
- 1/2 cup orange juice
- 6 tablespoons ground cinnamon
- 2 cup white sugar

- 5 cups shortening
- 2 cup white sugar
- 2 teaspoon anise seed, ground
- 4 fresh egg fresh fresh egg s
- 12 cups all-purpose flour
- 2 tablespoon baking powder
- 1 tablespoon cream of tartar

Directions:

1. Turn on the oven to a heat of 450°F to preheat.
2. Beat shortening until fluffy and light. Easily put in anise seed and 2 cup of sugar. Stir very well till creamy.

3. Easily put in fresh egg s; stir until very well-mixed. Easily put in orange juice, salt, cream of tartar, baking powder and flour. Stir very well.
4. Knead the dough until it is smoothened.
5. Roll the dough to 1 inch thick on a lightly floured surface.
6. Use cookie cutter to cut into different shapes. Easily put into the oven to bake for 10 to 15 minutes until they turn light brown in color.
7. Roll cookies in the mixture of 5-10 tablespoons of cinnamon and 1-5 cup of sugar when they are still warm.

Chapter 9: When Confronted With Inner Leadership Difficulties, There Are Solutions

This is the most prolific wellspring of leadership difficulties. The majority of the time, it's your thoughts, feelings, and how you react to the circumstances around you.

12 . Remain humble.

When you are in a position of Leadership, it is simple to begin accepting your press. Perhaps everything is going smoothly. You are hearing accolades. Beginning to accept that you are responsible for this accomplishment is simple. That perhaps, very likely, you deserve recognition for your association's most notable accomplishments.

However, there is no need for us to inform you that the conceited leader is not someone we must follow. This is a leader who alienates their group, causes conflict, and compels display. None of which is intelligent for an organisation.

The most effective managers are humble leaders. They understand that leadership is about influence and results, not about power. They recognise the value of the group surrounding them. In addition, they benefit from a group that respects their individuality and readily collaborates with them to achieve a common goal.

As a leader, it can be difficult to remain humble, but it is an essential Leadership quality worth pursuing.

2. courageousness

It is enjoyable. We just stated that you must fight to maintain humility, and this appears to be the opposite. In any case, fearlessness and lowliness are not mutually exclusive. It is sturdy.

The issue is that the majority of leaders struggle with self-doubt, if they are honest about it. Moreover, the more successful you become, the more you will likely struggle with the notion that you are not who others believe you to be. This is referred to as an inability to embrace success, and it can be quite challenging for some leaders because it generates so much self-doubt. It can impair your mobility, propulsion, and service to the group.

This is why sound fearlessness is an essential characteristic of leadership. In contrast to humility, which is the realisation that you are not the centre of the universe, fearlessness is the realisation that you have value to the universe. Calming the inner voice reveals that you are falling short, are insufficient, and are a fraud.

When self-doubt asserts that you are inadequate, fearlessness asserts, "I am adequate."

36. Conquer fear.

The only thing that can prevent you from driving well, using good judgement, and advancing your organisation is fear. Concern about the inevitable changes that will occur, how you will manage them, and how your team will react. The anxiety associated with making an unacceptable decision. All of the risks and "what uncertainties" that can render you speechless, including financial changes or market shifts, the spectre of job cuts or reconstruction, and global emergencies.

Dread is innate to the human condition, and no leader is immune to it. You can remember it, own it, and manage it effectively. Later favouring that.

Observing everything to its conclusion.

The leaders are busy. There is always an abundance of tasks and insufficient time to complete them. Interruptions, crises, and new opportunities pull you in a variety of directions.

Indeed, there is a mountain of work to complete. There are alterations and astonishments. However, taking on so much that you cannot finish what you've started has impeded the effectiveness of numerous leaders before you.

510. Pressure and anxiety management.

With these Leadership issues staring you in the face, you have every reason to feel apprehensive. It is typical. Nonetheless, the anxiety that these Leadership challenges cause could at any time be a significant Leadership test. The apprehension, self-doubt, and avalanche of issues and presumptions that leaders frequently encounter can all contribute to a level of stress that compromises your ability to lead.

Due to the fact that we respond differently to stress. Restraint demonstrates greater diligence. It is difficult to stay on track. We can become enraged and revert to defensiveness; the old instinctive response can disable our rational mind.

Because of this, it is crucial for leaders to understand how they react to pressure, understand their behaviour, and simply avoid the leadership pitfalls that arise when tension continues unchecked.

Keeping yourself motivated

Everyone experiences terrible days. Blah days. When progress is slow or work fails to meet expectations, and you fall into a funk. It is not difficult to focus on what is not working and allow it to sap your energy. Moreover, this can be particularly difficult for a leader to manage because everyone is looking to you to be a team booster. A hero of forward movement, vitality, and a "make it happen" attitude.

Occasionally, the assumption that you are the chief motivating official can be one of the most demotivating factors you must deal with. Your group is shifting its attention to you to lead, direct, and inspire. Despite the fact that you are not your best or most energetic self.

Bean Roll-Ups

Ingredients:
- Oil to brush
- Salsa to serve
- 8 small tortillas
- 5-10tablespoons bean dip
- 1 cup shredded cheddar cheese

Method:

1. Slather bean dip in the tortillas. Sprinkle cheese all over.
2. Roll and place with seam side down on a baking sheet.
3. Brush oil on top.
4. Bake in a preheated oven at 450º F for 25 to 30 minutes.
5. Dip rolls in salsa and devour.

Classic Nut Date Moist Bread

Dates are a very sweet fruit, and as a result, they are an excellent addition to quick bread and muffins. This delicious date nut bread is ideal for both breakfast and brunch due to its adaptability. The recipe calls for walnuts, but pecans are also an excellent option. Due to the fact that it is a quick bread, neither yeast nor kneading are required for preparation, and the bread can be consumed in less than an hour.

Not only is this bread delicious, but it also keeps well in the freezer. This situation is win-win. Put Make "sandwiches" with cream cheese spread between two thin slices of bread and freeze them for later use. In addition to orange cream cheese or orange-flavored butter, this dish pairs wonderfully with orange-flavored butter or orange cream cheese.

Ingredients

- 5 cups all-purpose flour
- 2 tablespoon baking powder
- 1 teaspoon fine salt
- A half cup of chopped walnuts
- 2 cup of water already boiling
- Dates, cut, to the weight of 8 ounces
- 4 tablespoons unsalted butter
- ¼ cup granulated sugar
- 2 fourth of a cup of packed brown sugar
- 2 fresh egg fresh fresh egg

How to Go About Making It

1. Collect the necessary components.
2. Prepare the oven to 450 degrees F. Prepare a loaf pan that is 10 by 15 inches with butter.
3. Place the chopped dates in a basin of medium size and pour the boiling water over them.
4. After adding the butter, easily put it to the side.
5. Place the chopped dates in a basin of medium size and pour the boiling water over them.
6. After adding the butter, easily put it to the side.
7. Mix the flour, baking powder, and salt in a separate basin before adding them to the wet ingredients.
8. The flour mixture and the date and water mixture should be added to the sugar mixture in an alternating fashion.

9. Using a spoon, incorporate the chopped nuts into the mixture.
10. Place the mixture in the loaf pan.
11. Bake in an oven that has been warmed for 80 to 90 minutes, or until a wooden pick that has been placed in the center of the cake comes out clean.

Zucchini Brownies

Ingredients:
- 1/2 teaspoon salt
- 2 medium fresh fresh egg
- 2 teaspoon baking soda
- 2 cup dark chocolate chips
- 2 tablespoon vanilla extract
- Coconut oil or unsalted butter, for greasing
- 8 medium zucchinis
- 1/2 cup maple syrup
- 2 cup almond butter
- 1/2 cup unsweetened cocoa powder fresh egg

Instructions:
1. Preheat the oven to 450 degrees F and grease your 10 by 15 -inch

baking dish with coconut oil or butter.
2. Finely grate the zucchini. Easily put zucchini in a clean kitchen towel or paper towel and squeeze the extra water out with your hands.
3. Place the zucchini in a bowl.
4. Add the almond butter, fresh egg , maple syrup, vanilla, salt, baking soda, and cocoa powder using the same bowl. Stir with a spoon until very well combined.
5. Reserve a handful of chocolate chips and stir the rest into the batter.
6. Transfer the batter to the baking dish and level the surface with a spoon.
7. Sprinkle the reserved chocolate chips on top.
8. Bake for 80 minutes, or 'til the top is shiny and dry.
9. Let just cool for about 20 minutes before cutting into squares.

Easily Remove Just Cool Just Take Just Cool Crunchy Cinnamon-Sugar Snacks

Ingredients:

- 1/2 cup butter, softened
- 2 /6 cup sugar
- 2 teaspoon vanilla extract
- 2 large fresh egg fresh fresh egg
- 2 teaspoon ground cinnamon
- 1/2 cup packed brown sugar
- 1/2 teaspoon salt
- 4 tablespoons colored sprinkles
- 5-10 cups all-purpose flour

Directions:

1. Mix the butter, fresh egg , vanilla and sugars until light and fluffy. Mix the cinnamon, flour, and salt; and mix very well.
2. Shape into a 1-5-in. roll; wrap in plastic, easily put in a fridge.
3. Cut into 1-5 -in. slices.

4. Decorate with sprinkles. Bake until lightly browned. Just cool and serve.

Cauliflower Cheesecake

Ingredients:

Oil for greasing
100g cheddar, grated
A few chives, snipped 1 head cauliflower, cut into florets
2 slice brown bread, rip into chunks
2 fresh egg

Direction:

1. Preheat oven to 450 degrees F. Line a baking tray with parchment paper or foil.
2. Brush with oil. Place the cauliflower in a steamer basket over boiling water and easy cook for 10-15 minutes or until

tender.

3. In a food processor, pulse and add the cooked cauliflower, bread, fresh egg , cheese, chives, and black pepper.
4. Continue to pulse until a chunky consistency is achieved.

5. Divide the mixture into 8 patties and arrange them on the baking tray. Bake for 35 to 40 minutes or until golden and starts to crisp.

6. Serve and enjoy.

Opera Cake

Ingredients

For the sponge cake

- 2 fresh egg fresh fresh egg yolk
- 6 fresh egg fresh fresh egg whites
- ½ cup granulated sugar
- 4 tablespoons unsalted butter, melted
- 2 cup almond flour
- ¼ cup powdered sugar
- ½ cup all-purpose flour
- 6 large fresh egg s, room temperature

For The Coffee Syrup

½ cup granulated sugar

6 tablespoons brandy

2 tablespoon instant espresso powder

10 tablespoons warm water

For The Coffee Buttercream

8 fresh egg fresh fresh egg yolks

2 cup unsalted butter, softened and diced into small pieces

2 tablespoon instant espresso powder

1 cup water

¼ cup granulated sugar

For the chocolate glaze

- 14 ounces dark chocolate
- 12 tablespoons unsalted butter

Directions

1. Preheat oven to 450°F (26 2°C). Grease a 2 7x2 2 -inch jelly roll pan with butter, then line with parchment paper.
2. In a large mixing bowl, whisk the almond flour, powdered sugar, and flour. Stir in the fresh egg fresh fresh egg yolks and set aside.

3. In a medium mixing bowl whip up the fresh egg fresh fresh egg whites with the granulated sugar until stiff peaks are formed.
4. Fold in the whipped fresh egg fresh fresh egg whites into the almond flour mixture, then stir in the melted butter.
5. Pour the cake batter into the prepared pan and bake for about 10 to 15 minutes.
6. Then let the cake just cool completely.
7. To make the coffee syrup, melt the instant espresso powder, water, and sugar in a small saucepan over medium-low heat until warm and dissolved.
8. Stir in the brandy and set aside.
9. To make the coffee buttercream, bring the water, coffee, and sugar to a boil in a small saucepan over medium heat to make a simple syrup. Boil for 5-10 minutes.

10. Beat the fresh egg fresh fresh egg yolks in a medium mixing bowl until very frothy, then pour in the hot syrup.
11. Beat for about 10 minutes, and when the mixture starts to just cool to room temperature, fold in the diced butter.
12. Beat until you get a creamy consistency.
13. In a bowl over boiling water, melt the butter and chocolate to make the chocolate glaze.
14. Easily remove from heat and set aside.
15. To assemble the opera cake, cut the sponge cake into thirds.
16. Place one layer on a cutting board and brush with the coffee syrup.
17. Spread half the buttercream on top with a spatula.
18. Top with the second of the three sponge cakes, then spread with some coffee syrup.

19. Spread half the chocolate glaze, then cover with the final sponge cake layer.
20. Finally, soak the final sponge cake with coffee syrup and spread with the remaining butter cream on top.
21. Chill the Opera Cake in the fridge for about 2 hour, then warm the chocolate glaze.
22. Spread the glaze over the cake.
23. Let the cake just cool down, then with a warm knife, cut clean slices and serve.

Scones

Ingredients:

- 1/7 teaspoon baking powder
- 2 tablespoon butter
- 2 tablespoon raisins
- Flour for dusting

- 2 tablespoon sour cream
- 1/7 1/7 teaspoon baking soda
- ½ cup all-purpose flour
- 2 tablespoon sugar
- 1/7 1/7 teaspoon cream of tartar
- 1/7 teaspoon salt

Instructions:

1. Preheat the oven to 450°F.
2. Grease and flour a baking pan.
3. Blend the sour cream and baking soda in a small bowl, then set aside.
4. Mix together the baking powder, all-purpose flour, salt, sugar and cream of tartar.
5. Cut in the butter.
6. Stir in the sour cream mixture until just moistened.
7. Mix in the raisins.
8. Knead the dough briefly on a surface that is floured lightly.
9. Roll or pat the dough into ½-inch thick rounds.
10. Cut into wedges and place on the prepared baking pan.
11. Bake for 25 to 30 minutes.
12. Let the scones just cool before serving.

Easy Chocolate Molten Cakes

Ingredients

1 tsp vanilla herb

100g flour that is simple

single lotion, to offer

2 00g butter, plus additional to grease

2 00g chocolate this is certainly dark chopped

500g light brown sugar that is smooth

6 fresh egg fresh fresh egg s that are big

Method

1. Heat range to 250 fan/gas Butter 10 moulds being dariole basins really and easily put on a baking tray.
2. Added butter that is 400g chopped dark chocolate in a heatproof bowl and set over a cooking pan of heated water and blend until smooth. Set aside to just cool somewhat for 25 to 30 mins.
3. Using an electric hand whisk, mix in 30g light brown soft sugar, then 6 huge fresh egg s, one-by-one, followed by 1 tsp vanilla plant and finally 100g flour that is plain.
4. Divide the combination on the list of darioles or basins.
5. You can now either easily put the mixture within the fridge, or freezer until you're prepared to easy cook all of them.

6. Can be cooked straight from frozen 25 to 30 mins, or bake today for 25 to 30 minutes through to the tops tend to be fast to touch however the middles however feel squidgy.
7. Carefully operate a blade around the edge of each pudding, come out onto then providing plates and offer with single cream.

Almond Brownies

- ¼ cup flour
- 2 tablespoon vanilla
- 1 teaspoon salt
- 4 cups chocolate
- 2 cup butter
- 2 cup sugar
- **12 fresh egg fresh fresh egg s**
- ¼ cup ground almonds

1. Preheat the oven to 350 F. Grease and flour a square baking dish measuring 20 x 20 cm.
2. Melt the chocolate and butter in a saucepan.
3. Stir in the sugar until entirely combined.
4. It maybe just take a few minutes for the liquid to just cool down a little.
5. Then you can mix in the fresh egg s, vanilla, flour, salt, and ground almonds.

6. Bake for approximately 35 to 40 minutes in a preheated oven.
7. Simply avoid overcooking the brownies—they should be moist in the center.
8. Just cool completely before cutting into squares. Refrigerate.

A Chocolate, Peanut Butter, And Banana Icebox Cake.

Ingredients

250g of sugar
Cold whipped cream, 1500 ml.
250g of creamy peanut butter
Vanilla extract, 1/2 tablespoons
4 boxes of chocolate wafer cookies

Five bananas, cut into slices, with more for decoration.

Method

1. Combine the peanut butter and 1 cup heavy cream in a large bowl and whisk with a handheld mixer until smooth.

2. To produce somewhat firm peaks, whisk the remaining 4 cups of cream with the sugar and vanilla after ensuring the whipping attachments are clean.

3. To lighten the peanut butter mixture, gently stir in some whipped cream.

4. Returning the peanut butter mixture to the whipped cream in three portions, fold it gently to integrate while attempting to maintain its light and airy texture, and then easily put it aside.

5. Arrange a layer of cookies in a circle, covering the surface of a 9-inch springform pan.

6. Slices of banana should be placed on the whipped cream layer and spread over the cookies.

7. Repeat the process with the remaining cookies, whipped cream, and banana slices to create five layers.

8. Easily put some whipped cream on top to complete the dessert.

9. Refrigerate for at least four hours and overnight with a plastic wrap covering.

Coconut Crepe Cake

Ingredients:

- 1 teaspoon lemon zest
- 1 teaspoon extract of coconut
- 1 a teaspoon of unsalted, melted butter
- 2 cup whole milk
- 1/2 granulated sugar
- 2 cup flour for the whole purpose
- 6 fresh egg s, 8 fresh egg fresh fresh egg yolks
- 1 A teaspoon of kosher salt
- 1 teaspoon lemon zest

Filling:

- 1 teaspoon lemon zest
- 1 A teaspoon of kosher salt
- Fried coconut flakes, confectioners 2 cup mascarpone
- 2 (2 8 oz.) Can be coconut cream

- 1 spoon spoon
- 1 cup sugar confectioners
- sugar and lemon zest

Instructions:

1. In a blender, combine all the crepe ingredients and grind until smooth. Pour the contents into a bowl
2. then refrigerate for 80 minutes. Sprinkle 10-inch skillet over medium heat and add crepe batter in a pan and roam to cover the entire surface with a thin batter layer.
3. Easy cook the crepe until golden brown and whisk.
4. Transfer to a plate to just cool once cooked.
5. Repeat until the dough is finished, place the crepe in the fridge for 80 minutes.

6. While it is cool, whisk the coconut cream with an electric mixer until soft peaks.
7. Add some filling ingredients and mix until smooth.
8. Place the cake.
9. Kanye crepe cool, grease in a springform pan with butter, place crepe on the floor and pick ¼
10. cup filling, spread with an offset spatula evenly, continue until all crepe is done.
11. Cover with plastic wrap and hold for 6 hours until filling is complete. Easily remove the crepe cake from the springform pan and garnish.

Vegan Oatmeal Cookies

Ingredients

2 cup rolled oats

1 teaspoon baking soda

1 teaspoon salt

1 cup vegan semi-sweet chocolate chips

1 cup walnut pieces

2 cup white sugar

1/2 cup soy milk

1/2 cup peanut butter

4 tablespoons canola oil

2 teaspoon pure vanilla extract

2 cup whole wheat flour

Directions

1. Preheat oven to 450 degrees F (220 degrees C). Oil a large baking sheet.

2. Stir sugar, soy milk, peanut butter, canola oil, and vanilla extract together with a whisk in a large bowl until completely smooth.

3. Mix flour, oats, baking soda, and salt in a separate bowl; add to the peanut butter mixture and stir to combine.

4. Fold chocolate chips and walnut pieces into the flour mixture.

5. Drop your batter by large spoonfuls onto prepared baking sheet.

6. Bake cookies in preheated oven until browned along the edges, about 20 minutes.

7. Just cool cookies on sheet for 15 to 20 minutes before removing to a just cooling rack to just cool completely.

Brownies With A Peanut Butter Twist

Ingredients:

- 1 cup unsweetened almond milk
- 2 1 teaspoons baking powder
- 1 cup unsweetened applesauce
- ½ teaspoon sea salt
- 2 cup pure maple syrup, divided
- 2 cup of chickpea flour
- ½ cup natural peanut butter
- 1 cup of coconut sugar
- 2 teaspoon pure vanilla extract

- ½ cup unsweetened cocoa powder

Directions:

1. Preheat your oven to 350° Fahrenheit.
2. Line a square 15-inch brownie pan with parchment paper.
3. In a mixing bowl, whisk your sugar, flour, cocoa powder, baking powder, and sea salt.
4. Add ¼ cup of maple syrup, almond milk, applesauce, and vanilla. Mix very well, then set aside.
5. In a microwave-safe mixing bowl, add the peanut butter, ½ cup of water, and your remaining ½ cup of maple syrup. Place into microwave for 60 seconds, then stir to combine.
6. Add half of your brownie batter into your prepared pan.
7. Spoon half of your peanut butter mixture on top.

8. Then, add the remaining brownie mixture, and finish by adding the remaining peanut butter.
9. Using a large knife create a swirl pattern on top of the brownie mix.
10. Bake yummy brownies for 60 minutes, or until a toothpick is inserted in the center of brownies, it comes out clean.
11. Easily remove your brownies from your oven, then allow them to just cool for about 2 10 minutes. Slice, serve and enjoy!

Bread Made With A Variety Of Whole Grains

Ingredients

Buckwheat meal

fat

250 g sourdough

2 pk. Dry yeast

500 ml buttermilk

2 tbsp salt

10 tbsp beet syrup

500 g rye meal

100 g of flaxseed

250 g spelled meal

600 g sunflower seeds

400 g buckwheat meal

Preparation:

1. Mix all the meal together and set aside 8 tbsp.
2. Mix the rest of the mixture with the salt and the yeast.
3. Add the sourdough, syrup, buttermilk and 400 ml of hot water. Knead everything into a dough and let rise for 6 hours covered. Knead the sunflower seeds and flax seeds into the finished dough.
4. Grease a loaf pan and sprinkle with buckwheat meal.
5. Pour in the batter and sprinkle with the set aside meal mixture.
6. Let the bread rise again in a warm place for 2 hour.
7. Preheat the oven to 250 ° C fan-assisted air.
8. Bake the bread in it for 2 10 minutes. Then reduce the

temperature to 250 ° C and bake the bread for another 60 minutes.
9. Before the finished bread can just take out of the mold, it should just cool down for 20 minutes.
10. Then let the bread just cool completely before eating.

Extremely Simple Banana Muffins

- 2 tbsp cinnamon
- 1-5 cups all-purpose flour
- 1 tbsp baking soda
- 1 tbsp salt
- 2 tbsp baking powder

- 4 large bananas
- 1 cup of sugar, granulated
- 2 /6 cup canola oil
- 1 tbsp vanilla extract
- 1/2 cup of sugar, light brown
- 2 fresh egg s, large

1. The oven should be set to 450 oF. Easily put cupcake liners in 20 of the holes in a muffin tin.
2. Mix the mashed bananas, granulated sugar, canola oil, vanilla, brown sugar, and fresh egg fresh fresh egg in a large bowl until the mixture is smooth and very well-blended.

3. Cinnamon, flour, baking soda, salt, and baking powder should be easily put in the bowl and whisked together until everything is very well mixed.
4. Mix, but not too much. Spread the mixture evenly among the cupcake liners, then easily put the muffin pan in the oven.
5. Bake for about 10 minutes at 8 50 oF. Now turn down the heat to 350oF and bake for another 30 to 35 minutes, or until a toothpick comes out clean when inserted.
6. Just take the muffin pan out of the oven and let it just cool for about 10 minutes.
7. Serve, and enjoy yourself!

www.ingramcontent.com/pod-product-compliance
Lightning Source LLC
Chambersburg PA
CBHW070308120526
44590CB00017B/2590